Moulay Hfid Youssoufi
Zineb Hakkou
Hicham Elmsellem

Pharmacology and Drug Toxicology

Moulay Hfid Youssoufi
Zineb Hakkou
Hicham Elmsellem

Pharmacology and Drug Toxicology

Deciphering the Secrets of Their Effects and Risks

ScienciaScripts

Imprint

Any brand names and product names mentioned in this book are subject to trademark, brand or patent protection and are trademarks or registered trademarks of their respective holders. The use of brand names, product names, common names, trade names, product descriptions etc. even without a particular marking in this work is in no way to be construed to mean that such names may be regarded as unrestricted in respect of trademark and brand protection legislation and could thus be used by anyone.

Cover image: www.ingimage.com

This book is a translation from the original published under ISBN 978-620-6-70394-5.

Publisher:
Sciencia Scripts
is a trademark of
Dodo Books Indian Ocean Ltd. and OmniScriptum S.R.L publishing group

120 High Road, East Finchley, London, N2 9ED, United Kingdom
Str. Armeneasca 28/1, office 1, Chisinau MD-2012, Republic of Moldova, Europe
Printed at: see last page
ISBN: 978-620-7-22017-5

Copyright © Moulay Hfid Youssoufi, Zineb Hakkou, Hicham Elmsellem
Copyright © 2024 Dodo Books Indian Ocean Ltd. and OmniScriptum S.R.L publishing group

Pharmacology and Toxicology of
Medicines

Deciphering the Secrets of Their Effects and Risks

Pharmacology and Toxicology of Medicines
Deciphering the Secrets of Their Effects and Risks

Introduction

When we take a drug to alleviate our ailments or treat a disease, we are often aware of its beneficial effects. However, we may be less familiar with the complex mechanisms behind these effects and the potential risks associated with their use. This is where pharmacology and toxicology come in.

Pharmacology and toxicology are two closely related disciplines that study the interactions of chemical substances with living organisms. Pharmacology focuses on the effects of drugs on the body, including their absorption, distribution, metabolism and elimination, as well as their mechanisms of action. Toxicology, on the other hand, examines the adverse effects of chemical substances on health, whether they are present in drugs, industrial chemicals or the environment.

In this first part of our book, we explore the fundamentals of pharmacology and toxicology. We'll start with an in-depth introduction to these two disciplines, highlighting their importance in our understanding of drugs and their effects. We'll look at the fundamentals of pharmacokinetics and pharmacodynamics, which describe respectively how a drug behaves in the body and how it produces its effects.

In addition, we'll dive into the complex world of toxicology, examining key concepts such as dose-response, acute and chronic toxicity, as well as the different types of toxic effects. We'll also discuss the methods used to assess the risks associated with exposure to chemical substances, including preclinical and clinical studies, as well as the factors that can influence a drug's toxicity.

By understanding the basics of pharmacology and toxicology, we'll be better equipped to assess the benefits and risks of the drugs we take, and make informed decisions about our health. Get ready to dive into the fascinating world of drug interactions, molecular mechanisms and safety assessments as we explore the fundamentals of drug pharmacology and toxicology.

Part I: Fundamentals of pharmacology and toxicology

1. Introduction to drug pharmacology and toxicology

When we think of drug pharmacology and toxicology, we enter the fascinating field of interactions between chemical substances and the human body. Pharmacology and toxicology are essential disciplines for understanding how drugs act on our bodies and the risks associated with their use.

Pharmacology is the study of drugs, their composition, mode of action and effect on the human body. It encompasses the way drugs are absorbed, distributed, metabolized and eliminated by the body. Understanding these processes enables us to determine the appropriate dosage, optimize therapeutic effects and minimize side effects.

Toxicology, on the other hand, focuses on the study of the harmful effects of chemical substances on health. It assesses the toxic effects of drugs, as well as industrial chemicals, environmental toxins and other chemical agents. Toxicology examines the mechanisms by which these substances can damage organs, disrupt cellular functions and cause adverse effects.

In this first part of our book, we dive into the fundamentals of drug pharmacology and toxicology. We'll explore basic concepts such as bioavailability, which describes the amount of drug that reaches the bloodstream after administration, and drug distribution to target tissues in the body.

We will also cover pharmacodynamics, which studies the interactions between drugs and receptors present in the body, as well as the molecular mechanisms underlying their therapeutic effects. Understanding how drugs act on signalling pathways and biological processes gives us a better grasp of their desired and undesired effects.

In addition, we will explore the key concepts of toxicology, such as dose-response, acute and chronic toxicity, and the different types of toxic effects. We will examine the methods used to assess drug safety, including preclinical studies in animals and clinical trials in humans.

By understanding the basics of drug pharmacology and toxicology, we'll be able to critically apprehend the benefits and risks associated with their use. Prepare to plunge into a captivating journey through the mysteries of the interaction between drugs and the human body, and discover the essential foundations of drug pharmacology and toxicology.

2.   Fundamentals of pharmacokinetics and pharmacodynamics

Pharmacokinetics and pharmacodynamics are two essential disciplines for understanding how drugs interact with our bodies. Pharmacokinetics studies the processes of absorption, distribution, metabolism and elimination of drugs, while pharmacodynamics explores the interactions between drugs and biological targets, as well as the molecular mechanisms underlying their effects.

Pharmacokinetics :

Pharmacokinetics concerns the stages that drugs go through once they have been administered to the body. It begins with absorption, which is how the drug is absorbed into the bloodstream from its site of administration, whether by oral ingestion, intravenous injection or another route. Factors such as the drug's solubility, absorption surface and the presence of food may influence its rate and degree of absorption.

Once in the bloodstream, the drug is distributed to the body's various tissues and organs. Distribution is influenced by factors such as plasma protein binding, cell membrane permeability and tissue vascularization. Some drugs can also cross the blood-brain barrier to reach the central nervous system.

After distribution, drugs often undergo a process of metabolism in the liver, where they are converted into inactive or active metabolites. Liver enzymes play a key role in this biotransformation process. Some drugs may undergo first-pass metabolism reactions, meaning that they are partially or totally metabolized before reaching the systemic circulation.

Finally, drug elimination occurs mainly via the kidneys, through excretion in the urine. However, other elimination routes such as bile, lungs and sweat can also contribute to drug elimination.

Pharmacodynamics :

Pharmacodynamics is concerned with the effects of drugs on the body and the molecular mechanisms underlying these effects. It examines the interactions between drugs and receptors, enzymes, ion channels or other biological targets present in our bodies.

Drugs can act in a variety of ways, binding to receptors and modifying their activity, inhibiting or activating specific enzymes, or disrupting cellular processes. These interactions lead to a variety of biological responses, such as relieving symptoms, reducing inflammation, blocking nerve transmission or inhibiting cell growth.

Pharmacodynamics also studies dose-response relationships, which describe how the biological response varies according to the dose administered. This includes the desired therapeutic effect, as well as the adverse and toxic effects that can occur at high doses or in sensitive individuals.

By understanding the fundamental principles of pharmacokinetics and pharmacodynamics, we can better assess how drugs act in our bodies and how to adjust their use to optimize therapeutic benefits and minimize risks. This knowledge helps us to make informed decisions regarding the choice of drugs, appropriate dosages and necessary adjustments according to the individual characteristics of each patient.

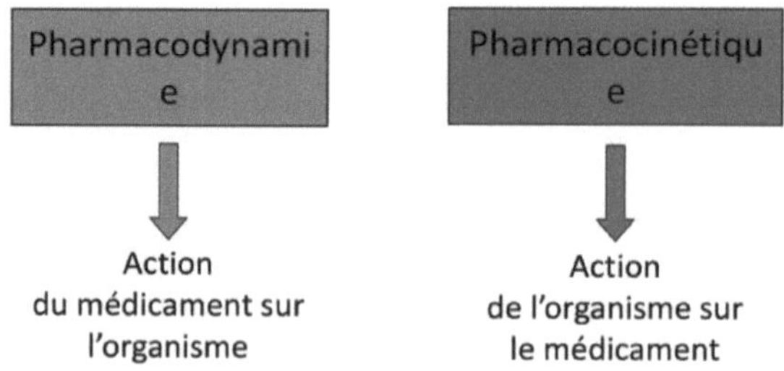

3. Key concepts in toxicology and risk assessment

Toxicology is an essential discipline for assessing the adverse effects of chemical substances, including drugs, on human health. It studies the mechanisms by which chemical substances can disrupt normal biological processes, cause toxic effects and potentially induce disease.

In this section, we explore the key concepts of toxicology and risk assessment associated with chemical exposure, with a focus on drugs.

- **Dose-response**: The concept of dose-response is fundamental to toxicology. It describes the relationship between the dose of a chemical substance administered and the biological response observed. The dose-response curve may be linear, follow a sigmoidal model or take other forms, depending on the substance and the effect observed. Toxicity can be classified into acute toxicity, which occurs after a single short-term exposure, and chronic toxicity, which occurs after repeated exposure over a prolonged period.

- **Factors influencing toxicity**: Several factors can influence the toxicity of a chemical substance, including the characteristics of the chemical itself, the route of exposure, the duration and frequency of exposure, and the individual characteristics of the exposed individual, such as age, gender, pre-existing health status and genetic susceptibility.

- **Types of toxic effects**: The toxic effects of chemical substances can be varied. They can include local effects at the site of exposure, such as skin irritation or lung damage, as well as systemic effects, such as effects on the nervous system, cardiovascular system, reproductive system, immune system or other organs. Some drugs may also have specific adverse effects, such as allergic reactions or teratogenic effects on embryonic development.

- **Risk assessment**: Toxicological risk assessment aims to estimate the potential hazards of a chemical substance and determine safe levels of exposure. This involves identifying toxicity thresholds, which represent exposure levels below which no harmful effects would be expected. Risk assessment also takes into account possible routes of exposure, frequency of exposure and sensitive populations.

- **Pre-clinical and clinical studies**: Before a drug is approved for use in humans, it undergoes pre-clinical studies in animal models to assess its toxicity, pharmacokinetics and pharmacodynamics. These studies provide crucial information for decisions concerning human clinical trials. Clinical trials evaluate the drug's efficacy and safety in patients.

By understanding the key concepts of toxicology and risk assessment, we are better equipped to evaluate the potential hazards associated with drug use, and to make informed decisions about their safe use. This knowledge enables us to ensure patient safety and optimize therapeutic benefits while minimizing the risks associated with chemical exposure.

Part II: Drug mechanisms of action

4. Drug interactions: synergies and antagonisms

When several drugs are taken simultaneously, it's important to understand how they may interact with each other. Drug interactions can result in synergistic effects, where drugs act in an enhanced way, or antagonistic effects, where they neutralize each other. This section will explore the different types of drug interactions and their implications.

- **Synergies** : Synergies occur when the combined effect of two drugs is greater than the sum of their individual effects. In some cases, two drugs with similar modes of action can produce a synergistic effect by acting on the same biological pathway. For example, the combination of an opioid analgesic with a non-opioid analgesic can lead to greater pain relief than the use of a single drug.

- **Antagonisms**: Antagonisms occur when the effect of one drug is reduced or cancelled by the presence of another drug. There are several types of antagonism, such as competitive antagonism, where drugs compete for the same receptors, or functional antagonism, where drugs act on opposite biological pathways. For example, the simultaneous use of an agonist and an antagonist at a receptor can lead to a diminished effect of the agonist.

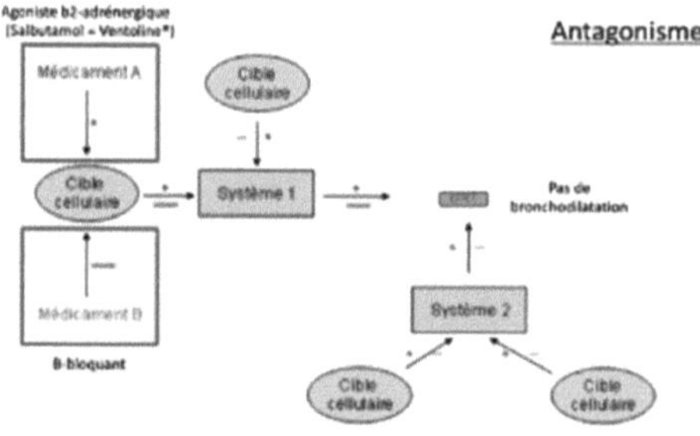

- **Pharmacokinetic interactions**: Drug interactions can also occur at the level of pharmacokinetics, i.e. drug absorption, distribution, metabolism and elimination. Some drugs can influence these processes, resulting in changes in the blood concentrations of other drugs. For example, one drug may inhibit a hepatic enzyme responsible for the metabolism of another drug, thereby increasing its plasma concentration and potentially its adverse effects.

- **Interactions with food and beverages**: It is also important to consider drug interactions with food and beverages. Certain foods and beverages can alter drug absorption or influence drug metabolism. For example, consumption of grapefruit juice can inhibit liver enzymes, thereby increasing the concentration of certain drugs in the body.

- **Importance of monitoring and communication**: Close monitoring of drug interactions is essential to minimize potential health risks. Healthcare professionals must be informed of all medications taken by a patient, including prescription, over-the-counter and herbal remedies. Clear communication between patient and healthcare professional is crucial to avoid unwanted drug interactions and adjust treatments accordingly.

By understanding drug interactions, whether synergistic or antagonistic, we can better manage polypharmacy and minimize health risks. Prudent drug use and proper monitoring can ensure safe and effective treatments, optimizing therapeutic outcomes while avoiding potential adverse effects.

5. Cellular targets: receptors, enzymes and ion channels

Drugs exert their therapeutic effects by interacting with specific targets within cells. These cellular targets include receptors, enzymes and ion channels, which play essential roles in the regulation of biological processes. Understanding these cellular targets in detail is crucial to understanding the mechanisms of drug action.

- **Receptors**: Receptors are proteins located on or inside cell surfaces. They act as signal receptors and are responsible for transmitting information within the cell in response to specific stimuli, such as neurotransmitters, hormones or drugs. Drugs can bind to these receptors, either by attaching directly to their binding site, or by altering their conformation. This interaction can activate or inhibit receptor function, triggering a cascade of intracellular signals and producing specific effects. For example, beta-blockers used to treat hypertension bind to beta-adrenergic receptors, thus blocking the stimulatory effects of catecholamines on the cardiovascular system.

- **Enzymes**: Enzymes are proteins that catalyze specific chemical reactions in the body. They are essential to many biological processes, such as nutrient metabolism, protein synthesis and cell signal transmission. Some drugs act by inhibiting or activating specific enzymes. Enzyme inhibitors bind to the target enzyme and interfere with its catalytic activity, thereby inhibiting the chemical reaction it catalyzes. For example, angiotensin-converting enzyme inhibitors (ACEIs) used to treat hypertension block the enzyme responsible for converting angiotensin I to angiotensin II, thereby reducing vasoconstriction and sodium retention.

- **Ion channels**: Ion channels are membrane proteins that regulate the selective passage of ions across cell membranes. They play a crucial role in transmitting electrical signals and maintaining ionic balance within cells. Some drugs act by modulating the activity of ion channels, thus affecting electrical processes and cellular functions. Drugs can block or open ion channels, thereby altering the flow of ions across cell membranes. For example, calcium channel blockers used to treat hypertension and heart disorders inhibit the calcium channels responsible for calcium entry into muscle cells, thereby reducing cardiac contractility and blood pressure.

It's important to note that some drugs can target several cellular targets at once, and some drugs can have effects on different types of receptor, enzyme or ion channel. This interaction with specific cellular targets enables drugs to modulate biological processes and induce desired therapeutic effects.

Knowledge of the cellular targets of drugs is essential for understanding how they act and for predicting their effects on the body. This enables researchers and clinicians to design more specific drugs and optimize their clinical use. A better understanding of cellular targets contributes to more precise and effective drug therapy, offering treatment options tailored to individual diseases and patient needs.

6. Cell signaling pathways and synaptic transmission

Cell signaling pathways and synaptic transmission are essential processes for the communication and regulation of cellular functions. In the context of drug mechanisms of action, understanding these signaling pathways and synaptic transmission is crucial to understanding how drugs influence biological processes. This section will explore these key concepts and their importance in the mechanisms of drug action.

- **Cell signaling pathways**: Cell signaling pathways are complex intracellular communication systems that enable cells to detect and respond to environmental signals or signals from other cells. These pathways often involve the transmission of chemical signals, such as neurotransmitters, hormones or growth factors. When a chemical signal binds to a specific receptor on the cell surface, it triggers a cascade of intracellular reactions leading to specific responses, such as gene activation, modulation of enzyme activity or changes in membrane permeability.

Some drugs act by modulating cell signaling pathways. They can bind to receptors on the cell surface and influence biological responses by amplifying or inhibiting intracellular signals. For example, the selective serotonin reuptake inhibitors (SSRIs) used in the treatment of depression act by blocking serotonin reuptake, resulting in increased levels of serotonin in the synaptic cleft and modulation of associated signaling pathways.

- **Synaptic transmission**: Synaptic transmission is the process by which electrochemical signals are transmitted between neurons at synapses. Synapses are specialized junctions between neurons where chemical signals, called neurotransmitters, are released by a presynaptic cell and bind to specific receptors on a postsynaptic cell. This interaction between neurotransmitters and receptors triggers electrical or chemical responses in the postsynaptic cell, enabling the transmission of information from one neuron to another.

Some drugs act by modulating synaptic transmission. For example, selective serotonin reuptake inhibitor (SSRI) antidepressants increase serotonin levels in synapses, which in turn strengthens synaptic transmission and can improve depressive symptoms. Other drugs, such as the benzodiazepines used to treat anxiety, act by potentiating the action of the inhibitory neurotransmitter GABA (gamma-aminobutyric acid) at synapses.

Understanding cell signaling pathways and synaptic transmission is key to understanding how drugs modify biological processes and produce therapeutic effects. By specifically targeting these pathways and mechanisms, drugs can regulate cellular responses, restore chemical balance or compensate for dysfunctions associated with certain pathological conditions. A thorough understanding of these mechanisms enables researchers and clinicians to design more targeted drugs and optimize their clinical use for optimal therapeutic results.

Part III: Drug classes and their effects

In this chapter, we explore the different classes of drugs and their effects on the human body. Medicines play an essential role in the treatment of illnesses and medical conditions, and their appropriate use can improve patients' quality of life. Understanding the different classes of drugs and their mechanisms of action is crucial for healthcare professionals and patients alike.

We'll look at the main drug groups, such as analgesics, antibiotics, antihypertensives, antidepressants, anti-inflammatories, anticoagulants, antihistamines and many others. Each drug class has specific properties that target different body systems and treat specific conditions.

The study of these drug classes will include an exploration of their mechanisms of action, medical indications, therapeutic effects and possible side effects. We will also stress the importance of medical consultation and of taking medication only under the supervision of a qualified health professional.

It's essential to recognize that medications can have varying effects on different people due to factors such as age, weight, gender, medical history and other medications taken simultaneously. Therefore, a thorough knowledge of drug classes and their effects is necessary to avoid harmful interactions and adverse reactions.

By exploring drug classes and their effects, we aim to provide readers with a solid knowledge base for safe and effective medication use. Drug education is essential for responsible use, enabling patients to make informed decisions in collaboration with their healthcare professionals.

It should be noted that this chapter is not intended to replace individual medical advice. We strongly encourage readers to consult their healthcare professional for specific information regarding their medical conditions and prescribed medications.

By delving into drug classes and understanding their effects, we hope to contribute to a better understanding and use of medicines, with the ultimate aim of improving health and well-being for all.

7. Central nervous system drugs: analgesics, tranquilizers, antidepressants, etc.

In this detailed section on central nervous system drugs, we'll explore in depth the different drug classes and their specific effects. Let's start with analgesics.

- **Analgesics**: Analgesics are drugs used to relieve pain, whether acute or chronic. There are two main categories of analgesics: opioid analgesics and non-opioid analgesics.

  ❖ Opioid analgesics: Opioids, such as morphine, oxycodone and fentanyl, work by binding to opioid receptors in the central nervous system, blocking the transmission of pain signals. These drugs are generally used to treat severe pain, such as that associated with cancer, serious injury or major surgery. However, they can lead to dependence and side effects such as drowsiness, constipation and respiratory depression.

  ❖ Non-opioid analgesics: Non-opioid analgesics, such as ibuprofen, acetaminophen (paracetamol) and aspirin, work by inhibiting the enzymes responsible for producing inflammatory chemicals in the body, thereby reducing pain and inflammation. These drugs are commonly used to treat mild to moderate pain, such as headaches, muscle aches and joint pains. They generally have fewer side effects than opioid analgesics, but can cause gastrointestinal disorders and liver damage when used in high doses or for long periods.

- **Tranquilizers (Anxiolytics)**: Tranquilizers, also known as sedatives or anxiolytics, are used to treat anxiety, sleep disorders and mood disorders. They work by increasing the activity of the inhibitory neurotransmitter gamma-aminobutyric acid (GABA) in the brain, producing a calming effect and reducing anxiety.

  ❖ Benzodiazepines: Benzodiazepines, such as diazepam, lorazepam and alprazolam, are the most commonly prescribed tranquilizers. They work by enhancing GABA transmission in the brain, which reduces neuronal excitability and calms anxiety. Benzodiazepines are generally prescribed for short-term use, as they can lead to dependence and excessive sedation.

  ❖ Non-benzodiazepine medications: There are also other anxiolytic medications, such as buspirone and specific antidepressants with anxiolytic action, which can be used to treat anxiety without the dependence risks associated with benzodiazepines.

- **Antidepressants**: Antidepressants are used to treat mood disorders such as major depression, anxiety disorders and obsessive-compulsive disorders. There are several classes of antidepressants, each targeting different neurotransmitters in the brain.

- ❖ Selective serotonin reuptake inhibitors (SSRIs): SSRIs, such as fluoxetine, sertraline and escitalopram, increase serotonin levels in the brain by inhibiting its reuptake, thereby improving mood and reducing depressive symptoms. They are also used to treat anxiety disorders.

- ❖ Serotonin and norepinephrine reuptake inhibitors (SNRIs): SNRIs, such as venlafaxine and duloxetine, work by inhibiting the reuptake of serotonin and norepinephrine, two neurotransmitters involved in mood regulation. They are often prescribed for major depression and generalized anxiety disorder.

- ❖ Monoamine oxidase inhibitors (MAOIs): MAOIs, such as phenelzine and tranylcypromine, inhibit the activity of the enzyme monoamine oxidase, resulting in increased levels of serotonin, norepinephrine and dopamine. They are less commonly prescribed due to their potentially dangerous interactions with certain foods and drugs, which can cause a dangerous increase in blood pressure.

- **Antipsychotics**: Antipsychotics are used to treat psychotic disorders such as schizophrenia and bipolar disorder. They work by blocking dopamine receptors in the brain, reducing psychotic symptoms such as hallucinations, delusions and thought disorders.

- ❖ Typical antipsychotics: Typical antipsychotics, such as chlorpromazine and haloperidol, were the first drugs developed to treat schizophrenia. They tend to cause more neurological side effects, such as tremors and involuntary movements.

- ❖ Atypical antipsychotics: Atypical antipsychotics, such as olanzapine, risperidone and quetiapine, have emerged more recently. Their efficacy is similar to that of typical antipsychotics, but they have fewer neurological side effects. However, they can lead to weight gain and metabolic problems.

- **Mood stabilizers**: Mood stabilizers are used to treat bipolar disorder, characterized by alternating manic and depressive episodes. They help stabilize mood and prevent extreme fluctuations.

- ❖ Lithium: Lithium is the most commonly used mood stabilizer. Its exact mechanism of action is not fully understood, but it is thought to alter the levels of certain neurotransmitters in the brain. Lithium requires close monitoring of blood levels, as high levels can be toxic, while insufficient levels can be ineffective.

- ❖ Other mood stabilizers: Other drugs, such as valproate, carbamazepine and lamotrigine, may also be used as mood stabilizers, depending on the patient's specific needs.

It's important to stress that central nervous system medications must be prescribed and monitored by a qualified healthcare professional. Each class of medication has specific indications, potential side effects and precautions for use. Regular medical follow-up is essential to adjust doses, assess efficacy and minimize side effects.

8. Cardiovascular drugs: antihypertensives, anticoagulants, antiarrhythmics, etc.

In this detailed section on cardiovascular medications, we'll explore the different classes of drugs used to treat conditions related to the cardiovascular system. These drugs are essential for the management of conditions such as high blood pressure, heart rhythm disorders, coronary heart disease and stroke. Here are some of the main classes of cardiovascular drugs:

- **Antihypertensives**: Antihypertensives are used to treat hypertension, a condition characterized by high blood pressure. There are several classes of antihypertensives with different mechanisms of action:

- ❖ Angiotensin-converting enzyme (ACE) inhibitors: ACE inhibitors, such as enalapril and lisinopril, block the enzyme responsible for converting angiotensin I into angiotensin II, a substance that causes blood vessels to constrict. By inhibiting this enzyme, ACE inhibitors reduce vascular resistance and lower blood pressure.

- ❖ <u>Angiotensin II receptor blockers (ARBs)</u>: ARB IIs, such as losartan and valsartan, work by blocking angiotensin II receptors, preventing its vasoconstrictor action. This leads to vasodilation and lower blood pressure.

- ❖ <u>Beta-blockers</u>: Beta-blockers, such as propranolol and atenolol, block beta-adrenergic receptors in the heart, reducing heart rate and force of contraction. This lowers blood pressure and reduces the load on the heart.

- ❖ <u>Diuretics</u>: Diuretics, such as hydrochlorothiazide and furosemide, increase salt and water excretion by the kidneys, reducing blood volume and blood pressure.

- **Anticoagulants**: Anticoagulants are used to prevent blood clots and reduce the risk of thromboembolic complications, such as stroke and pulmonary embolism. The main classes of anticoagulants include:

- ❖ <u>Oral anticoagulants</u>: Oral anticoagulants, such as warfarin and newer oral anticoagulants (NACOs) such as apixaban and rivaroxaban, interfere with blood clotting by inhibiting coagulation factors. They require regular monitoring and may present drug interactions.

- ❖ <u>Heparin</u>: Heparin is an injectable anticoagulant that acts by inhibiting clot formation. It is often used in hospitals to prevent clot formation during surgery or in high-risk patients.

- **Anti-arrhythmics**: Anti-arrhythmics are used to treat cardiac rhythm disorders, such as atrial fibrillation, ventricular tachycardia and bradycardia. These drugs have specific mechanisms of action to normalize heart rhythm and maintain adequate cardiac function. The different classes of antiarrhythmic drugs include sodium channel blockers, beta-blockers, calcium channel blockers and potassium channel blockers.

- **Vasodilators**: Vasodilators are used to dilate blood vessels, thereby reducing vascular resistance and lowering blood pressure. They are used to treat hypertension and angina pectoris. Vasodilators may act by relaxing the smooth muscles of the blood vessels or by inhibiting contraction of the heart's muscle cells. Some common examples of vasodilators include nitroglycerin, calcium channel blockers and nitrate derivatives.

It is essential to emphasize that cardiovascular drugs must be prescribed and monitored by a qualified healthcare professional, as they can have drug interactions, side effects and require regular evaluation of treatment efficacy. Appropriate use and compliance with medical guidelines are crucial to controlling cardiovascular conditions and preventing potentially serious complications.

9. Respiratory drugs: bronchodilators, antihistamines, corticosteroids, etc.

- **Bronchodilators**: Bronchodilators are drugs used to open airways and facilitate breathing. They are widely used in the treatment of asthma, chronic bronchitis, COPD and other respiratory conditions. Bronchodilators work by relaxing the smooth muscles of the airways, enabling better air circulation. There are several types of bronchodilator:

❖ Short-acting beta-2 agonists: These drugs, such as salbutamol and terbutaline, are often used as inhalers to relieve acute symptoms such as airway constriction, cough and shortness of breath. They work by stimulating beta-2 receptors in airway muscles, leading to muscle relaxation and airway dilation.

❖ Long-acting beta-2 agonists: These drugs, such as formoterol and salmeterol, are used for prolonged relief of respiratory symptoms. They are often combined with inhaled corticosteroids for more effective control of asthma and COPD.

❖ Short- and long-acting anticholinergics: Anticholinergics, such as ipratropium and tiotropium, block the action of acetylcholine, a neurotransmitter that causes airway constriction. They are commonly used to reduce airway constriction and prevent muscle spasms.

- **Inhaled corticosteroids**: Inhaled corticosteroids are anti-inflammatory drugs used in the treatment of asthma and certain chronic obstructive pulmonary diseases. They work by reducing airway inflammation, thereby controlling symptoms and preventing exacerbations. Inhaled corticosteroids are generally used on a daily basis and must be taken regularly to achieve optimal inflammation control.

- **Antihistamines**: Antihistamines are drugs used to treat the symptoms of respiratory allergies, such as sneezing, nasal congestion and itching. They work by blocking the action of histamine, a chemical released during an allergic reaction. Antihistamines can be taken orally or as nasal sprays to relieve allergic symptoms.

- Leukotriene antagonists: Leukotriene antagonists are drugs that block the action of leukotrienes, inflammatory substances involved in allergic reactions and airway inflammation. They are used in the treatment of asthma and can be administered orally. Leukotriene antagonists help reduce airway inflammation and prevent asthma symptoms.

- Systemic corticosteroids: Systemic corticosteroids, such as prednisone, are used to treat severe exacerbations of asthma or other respiratory conditions. They have powerful anti-inflammatory effects and are administered orally or by injection.

It's important to stress that the use of respiratory medications should be guided by a qualified healthcare professional. Each drug has specific indications, potential side effects and precautions for use. Regular medical follow-up is essential to assess treatment efficacy, adjust doses if necessary and minimize side effects.

10.   Digestive system drugs: antacids, antiemetics, laxatives, etc.

- **Antacids**: Antacids are medications used to treat stomach acid disorders such as heartburn, acid reflux and indigestion. They work by neutralizing excess gastric acid in the stomach, thus relieving symptoms. Antacids may contain ingredients such as calcium carbonate, sodium bicarbonate, aluminum hydroxide and magnesium hydroxide. Some antacids may also form a protective layer over the stomach mucosa to reduce irritation.

- **Antiemetics**: Antiemetics are drugs used to prevent or relieve nausea and vomiting. They can be used in the treatment of nausea and vomiting caused by a variety of conditions, such as drug side effects, chemotherapy, pregnancy, motion sickness and gastrointestinal infections. Antiemetics may act by blocking serotonin receptors (5-HT3), dopamine receptors (D2) or neurokinin receptors (NK1) in the brain and intestine, thereby reducing the sensations of nausea and vomiting.

- **Laxatives**: Laxatives are medicines used to treat constipation by facilitating stool evacuation. There are several types of laxative with different mechanisms of action:

❖ Osmotic laxatives: These laxatives, such as lactulose and polyethylene glycol, work by increasing the amount of water in the intestines, which softens stools and facilitates their passage.

❖ Stimulant laxatives: These laxatives, such as senna and bisacodyl, stimulate muscle contractions in the intestines, promoting stool movement.

❖ Ballast laxatives: These laxatives, such as wheat bran and psyllium seeds, increase stool volume and stimulate intestinal movement.

❖ Lubricating laxatives: These laxatives, such as mineral oil, lubricate the stool, making it easier to pass.

❖ Stool softeners: These laxatives, such as docusate sodium, soften stools by facilitating the penetration of water into the intestines.

- **Anti-diarrheals**: Anti-diarrheals are drugs used to treat diarrhea by reducing intestinal motility and increasing water absorption in the intestines. They help normalize bowel movements and reduce the frequency of diarrhea episodes. Some anti-diarrheal agents, such as loperamide, slow intestinal movements, while others, such as bismuth subsalicylate, work by reducing inflammation in the intestine.

- **Antispasmodics**: Antispasmodics are drugs used to relieve spasms and cramps in the muscles of the intestine. They are often used to treat functional bowel disorders, such as irritable bowel syndrome. Antispasmodics work by relaxing the smooth muscles of the intestine, reducing abdominal pain and spasms.

It's important to stress that the use of these digestive system medications should be guided by a qualified healthcare professional. Each drug has specific indications, potential side effects and precautions for use. It's also essential to understand that these drugs are often used for short-term symptomatic relief, and that a proper medical evaluation is required to determine the underlying cause of digestive disorders and implement a targeted, appropriate treatment.

11. Endocrine drugs: hormones, antidiabetics, thyroid hormones, etc.

- **Thyroid hormones**: Thyroid hormones, such as thyroxine (T4) and triiodothyronine (T3), are essential for regulating metabolism, growth and development. Thyroid medications are used to treat thyroid disorders such as hypothyroidism (insufficient production of thyroid hormones) and hyperthyroidism (excessive production of thyroid hormones).

- ❖ Hypothyroidism: In the case of hypothyroidism, levothyroxine-containing drugs are prescribed to supplement thyroid hormone levels. Levothyroxine is a synthetic form of T4 thyroid hormone. It is administered orally and helps compensate for hormone deficiency and normalize metabolism.

- ❖ Hyperthyroidism: For hyperthyroidism, drugs such as methimazole and propylthiouracil are used to reduce excessive thyroid hormone production. These drugs block the action of the enzymes responsible for thyroid hormone production.

- **Antidiabetics**: Antidiabetics are used to treat diabetes, a disease characterized by chronically elevated blood sugar levels. There are several classes of antidiabetic drugs:

- ❖ Insulin: Insulin is a hormone produced by the pancreas that regulates blood sugar levels. In type 1 diabetes, where there is insufficient insulin production, insulin therapy is required to control blood sugar levels. In type 2 diabetes, oral or injectable drugs can be used to improve insulin sensitivity or stimulate insulin production by the pancreas.

- ❖ Biguanides: Drugs in the biguanide class, such as metformin, are commonly used to treat type 2 diabetes. They work by reducing glucose production by the liver and improving glucose utilization by cells.

- ❖ <u>Hypoglycemic sulfonamides</u>: These drugs, such as glipizide and glibenclamide, stimulate insulin secretion by the pancreas. They help lower blood sugar by increasing the amount of insulin available.

- ❖ <u>Alpha-glucosidase inhibitors</u>: These drugs, such as acarbose, work by inhibiting the enzyme responsible for breaking down complex carbohydrates in the intestine. This slows carbohydrate absorption, helping to control blood glucose levels after meals.

- **Steroid hormones**: Steroid hormones, such as corticosteroids, are used to treat a variety of endocrine, inflammatory and autoimmune conditions. Corticosteroids, such as prednisone and dexamethasone, are used to suppress inflammation, modulate the immune response and treat conditions such as asthma, arthritis and autoimmune diseases.

- **Growth hormones**: Growth hormones, such as somatropin, are used to treat growth hormone deficiency in children and adults. These drugs stimulate growth, promote muscle and bone development, and can be used to treat conditions such as growth retardation or Turner syndrome.

It's important to stress that endocrine medications must be prescribed and monitored by a qualified healthcare professional. Each class of medication has specific indications, potential side effects and precautions for use. Dosage and frequency of administration may vary according to the condition being treated and the patient's individual needs. Regular medical follow-up is essential to assess treatment efficacy and adjust doses if necessary.

Part IV: Applied pharmacology and toxicology

This section, entitled "Applied Pharmacology and Toxicology", explores the fascinating field of drugs and their interaction with the human body. Pharmacology is the study of the effects of drugs on the body, while toxicology focuses on the harmful effects of toxic substances. Understanding these areas is essential to ensure the safe and effective use of medicines, as well as to assess the risks associated with exposure to potentially harmful substances.

This chapter examines the fundamentals of pharmacology and toxicology, as well as the different classes of drugs and their effects on the human body. We will also explore methods of drug administration, mechanisms of action, drug interactions and considerations related to the efficacy and safety of pharmacological treatments.

We'll also look at the importance of clinical research and drug evaluation in guaranteeing quality, efficacy and safety. Pharmacovigilance, which involves monitoring and reporting adverse drug reactions, will also be discussed.

With regard to toxicology, we will examine the different routes of exposure to toxic substances, methods of detection and risk assessment, and strategies for preventing and managing poisoning.

This chapter aims to provide an in-depth understanding of drugs, their clinical use, mechanisms of action and toxicological implications. By acquiring this knowledge, readers will be able to make informed decisions about drug use, minimize associated risks and promote health and well-being.

12.Pharmacogenetics: the impact of genetic variations on drug response

Pharmacogenetics is a fast-growing field that studies the influence of genetic variations on individual drug response. It enables us to understand why certain individuals may react differently to a given drug, in terms of efficacy and tolerance, due to their genetic differences. This knowledge makes it possible to personalize drug treatments according to each patient's genetic characteristics, thereby improving therapeutic results and minimizing adverse effects.

Genetic variations can have an impact on many aspects of drug response, including absorption, distribution, metabolism and elimination of drugs in the body. Some genetic variations can result in altered enzyme activity, which can influence the rate at which a drug is metabolized. For example, cytochrome P450 is a family of enzymes involved in the metabolism of many drugs. Genetic variations in the genes encoding these enzymes can lead to faster or slower metabolism of drugs, with important implications for their efficacy and toxicity.

A well-known example of pharmacogenetics is the CYP2D6 enzyme, which is responsible for the metabolism of many drugs, including some antidepressants and antipsychotics. Individuals can exhibit genetic variations in the CYP2D6 gene, which can lead to different metabolic phenotypes, such as fast metabolizers, slow metabolizers or non-metabolizers. These metabolic differences can influence the plasma concentration of a given drug, thus affecting its efficacy and tolerability.

Pharmacogenetics is also relevant to anticancer drugs, where specific genetic variations may be associated with tumor response or treatment toxicity. For example, the identification of certain genetic mutations in tumors can guide the choice of a specific targeted therapy, improving treatment efficacy and patient survival.

Pharmacogenetics can be applied at various levels. In some cases, prior genetic testing can be carried out to identify specific genetic variations that may influence response to a given drug. This information can then be used to personalize treatment, by adjusting doses or choosing more suitable therapeutic alternatives.

However, it is important to note that pharmacogenetics should not be considered as a single approach to clinical decision-making. It needs to be integrated into a more comprehensive approach, taking into account other factors such as the patient's general state of health, drug interactions and the specific clinical features of the disease.

In conclusion, pharmacogenetics opens up exciting new perspectives in pharmacotherapy, enabling a more individualized approach to drug treatment. By understanding how genetic variations influence drug response, healthcare professionals can optimize the efficacy and safety of treatments, improving therapeutic outcomes for every patient.

13.Medicines for special populations: children, the elderly, pregnant women, etc.

This chapter examines medication use in special populations, such as children, the elderly and pregnant women. These population groups have unique physiological characteristics and health needs that require a specific approach to medication. Understanding the special considerations associated with medication use in these populations is essential to ensure safe and effective management. Here's a detailed section on medication use in special populations:

- **Medicines in children**: Medication use in children presents unique challenges due to physiological differences, ongoing growth and development. Children may have different drug absorption, distribution, metabolism and elimination than adults. Therefore, it is essential to adapt doses according to each child's age, weight and individual characteristics.

- ❖ Adapted formulations: Children's medicines are often formulated as liquids, chewable tablets, syrups or suspensions to facilitate administration and allow doses to be adjusted according to the child's body weight. Specific studies are carried out to assess the safety and efficacy of medicines in children.

- ❖ Adverse drug reaction assessment: Children may be more sensitive to adverse drug reactions. Close monitoring of potential adverse effects is essential to ensure the safety of drugs used in children.

- ❖ Pediatric studies: In many countries, regulations have been introduced to encourage specific clinical studies in children, to ensure that drugs used in this population are safe and effective.

- **Medication in the elderly**: The elderly have age-related physiological changes that may influence drug response. Factors such as decreased renal and hepatic function, reduced muscle mass and concomitant diseases must be taken into account when prescribing drugs to the elderly.

- ❖ Polypharmacy: The elderly are often treated with multiple medications due to the presence of several chronic conditions. Polypharmacy can increase the risk of drug interactions and adverse effects. Regular assessment of current medications and simplification of treatment regimens may be necessary to minimize risks.

- ❖ <u>Preventing falls</u>: Certain medications used in the elderly can increase the risk of falls, due to their effects on balance and coordination. It is important to assess the risks associated with the use of these medications, and to adapt treatments accordingly.

- ❖ <u>Sensitivity to adverse effects</u>: Elderly people may be more sensitive to adverse drug reactions due to reduced renal and hepatic function, as well as changes in receptor sensitivity. Close monitoring for adverse effects is essential.

- **Medicines for pregnant women**: Prescribing medication to pregnant women is a delicate area, as drugs can have effects on the developing fetus. In many cases, it is preferable to avoid the use of drugs during pregnancy, particularly during the first trimester, when the fetal organs and systems are forming. However, there may be situations where the potential benefit of treatment outweighs the potential risk to the fetus.

- ❖ <u>Risk-benefit assessment</u>: Before prescribing a drug to a pregnant woman, it is essential to carefully weigh the potential risks to the fetus against the benefits of treatment for the mother.

- ❖ <u>Safe drugs during pregnancy</u>: Some drugs, such as certain antibiotics and analgesics, are considered relatively safe during pregnancy, and can be used if necessary. However, each situation must be evaluated individually.

- ❖ <u>Monitoring and follow-up</u>: Pregnant women taking medication should be closely monitored for any potential adverse effects on the fetus or mother. It is important to communicate regularly with health-care professionals to assess the efficacy and safety of treatment.

It is crucial to note that the use of drugs in special populations must be guided by qualified and informed healthcare professionals. An individual assessment of each patient, taking into account factors such as age, health status and specific characteristics, is essential to ensure the safe and effective use of medicines.

14. Drug toxicology: adverse effects, overdose, poisoning

Introduction: Drug toxicology is a discipline dedicated to the study of adverse effects, overdose and intoxication associated with the use of drugs. Although drugs are designed to treat, alleviate or prevent disease, there are potential risks when they are used inappropriately or when there is excessive exposure. This chapter looks in detail at the various aspects of drug toxicology, including adverse effects, overdose and intoxication, to provide a better understanding of the harmful consequences associated with drug use.

- **Adverse drug reactions**: Adverse drug reactions are harmful, undesired reactions that occur during normal drug use. They can vary in severity, from minor and temporary to severe and long-lasting. Some common side effects include nausea, headaches, skin rashes, gastrointestinal disorders, dizziness, sleep disturbances, etc. It is important to carefully monitor adverse effects when using medications and to report them to a healthcare professional if necessary. Some side effects may require discontinuation of the medication, while others can be managed with dosage adjustments or other medical interventions.

- **Drug overdose**: Drug overdose occurs when the administration of an excessive amount of medication exceeds recommended safety limits. This can happen accidentally, through dosage error, or intentionally, in the case of a suicide attempt. Overdosage can lead to serious, even life-threatening, adverse effects. Symptoms of overdose vary according to the drug involved, the dose ingested and individual sensitivity. They may include cardiovascular, respiratory, neurological, hepatic or renal disorders. In the event of an overdose, immediate medical intervention is required to assess the severity of the intoxication and take the necessary measures to minimize damage and treat symptoms. In severe cases, specific antidotes may be administered to counteract the drug's toxic effects.

- **Drug poisoning**: Drug poisoning can result from accidental exposure, misuse or attempted suicide. The drugs most commonly implicated in poisoning include analgesics, sleeping pills, antidepressants, benzodiazepines, opioid painkillers, anticoagulants, etc. Symptoms of drug intoxication vary according to the substance and dose ingested. They may include symptoms such as impaired consciousness, breathing difficulties, convulsions, heart problems, gastrointestinal problems, etc. In the event of drug intoxication, emergency medical care is required to assess the severity of exposure, administer appropriate treatment and monitor vital functions.

- **Poisoning prevention and management** : Preventing drug poisoning is essential to minimize health risks. This involves measures such as storing medicines safely out of the reach of children, taking medicines in accordance with instructions and prescribed dosages, consulting a healthcare professional before taking new medicines, and raising awareness of the potential dangers of self-medication. In the event of intoxication, management involves rapid and accurate assessment, supportive measures such as the administration of antidotes where necessary, and ongoing monitoring of the patient's condition.

Drug toxicology plays an essential role in understanding the adverse effects, overdoses and intoxications associated with drug use. A thorough knowledge of these aspects enables us to identify potential risks, prevent toxic incidents and provide adequate management in the event of intoxication. It is important that healthcare professionals and patients are aware of these risks, and work together to ensure the safe and appropriate use of medicines.

15. Drug monitoring and regulation: pharmacovigilance and marketing authorizations

Drug monitoring and regulation are essential elements in ensuring the safety and efficacy of medicines used in clinical practice. Pharmacovigilance and marketing authorization are key processes for monitoring adverse drug reactions and assessing the quality, efficacy and safety of medicines before they are marketed. This chapter looks in detail at these important aspects of drug monitoring and regulation.

Pharmacovigilance :

Pharmacovigilance is the process of continuously monitoring the adverse effects of medicines once they are on the market. Its main objective is to detect, assess, understand and prevent adverse reactions and safety problems associated with the use of medicines. Healthcare professionals, patients and drug manufacturers are encouraged to report suspected adverse reactions, whether known or new, to the relevant pharmacovigilance authority.

❖ <u>Collecting and evaluating adverse reaction reports</u>: Health authorities collect adverse reaction reports from a variety of sources, including healthcare professionals, patients, clinical trials and scientific literature. These reports are evaluated to determine the causality between the suspected drug and the reported adverse reaction.

❖ <u>Risk management</u>: Pharmacovigilance plays a key role in managing the risks associated with the use of medicines. On the basis of pharmacovigilance data, actions can be taken to minimize risks, such as modifying product information, implementing measures to restrict use, or withdrawing the drug from the market if the risks outweigh the benefits.

❖ <u>Information exchange</u>: Pharmacovigilance also involves sharing information between national and international health authorities, as well as between healthcare professionals and patients. This enables global monitoring of medicines and a better understanding of the potential risks associated with their use.

Marketing authorizations :

Before a drug can be marketed, it must go through a marketing authorization process. This procedure is designed to assess the quality, efficacy and safety of the drug, as well as its benefit-risk ratio, to ensure that it meets the appropriate regulatory standards. Marketing authorizations are issued by the relevant health authorities, such as the Agence nationale de sécurité du médicament et des produits de santé (ANSM) in France, or the Food and Drug Administration (FDA) in the United States.

❖ <u>Preclinical and clinical evaluation</u>: Before a drug is granted marketing authorization, it must undergo rigorous preclinical and clinical studies.

Preclinical trials evaluate the safety and efficacy of the drug in animal models, while clinical trials are conducted on human volunteers to assess the efficacy and safety of the drug under controlled conditions.

* ❖ <u>Marketing authorization file</u>: Drug manufacturers must submit a marketing authorization file containing data on the quality, safety and efficacy of the drug, as well as information on dosage, therapeutic indications and precautions for use. This dossier is evaluated by the health authorities, who then decide whether or not to grant marketing authorization.

* ❖ <u>Post-marketing surveillance</u>: Once a drug is on the market, its safety and efficacy continue to be monitored through pharmacovigilance. Post-marketing studies may also be carried out to evaluate the drug's widespread use and detect any safety problems not detected during clinical trials.

Drug monitoring and regulation play a crucial role in protecting public health, by ensuring that the medicines available on the market are safe, effective and of high quality. Pharmacovigilance enables the continuous monitoring of adverse drug reactions, while marketing authorizations ensure that

Part V: Future prospects and challenges

The "Future perspectives and challenges" chapter explores the emerging trends and challenges shaping the future of pharmacology and toxicology. As medical science continues to advance, new approaches, technologies and regulations are opening up new vistas and raising exciting challenges. This chapter examines recent developments and promising areas in these disciplines, as well as the obstacles they face.

- **Technological advances**: Technological advances are having a significant impact on pharmacology and toxicology. Tools such as genomics, proteomics, metabolomics and bioinformatics are enabling a deeper understanding of drug mechanisms of action, individual responses and toxicological risks. Advanced medical imaging techniques offer new opportunities for non-invasive assessment of drug efficacy and early detection of adverse effects. Advances in artificial intelligence and machine learning enable faster data analysis and interpretation, facilitating new drug discovery and treatment optimization.

- **Personalized medicine**: Personalized medicine is an emerging approach that aims to tailor medical treatments to individual patient characteristics, including genetic profile, biomarkers and environmental factors. This promising approach has the potential to improve treatment efficacy, reduce adverse effects and optimize clinical outcomes. Pharmacogenetics, which studies the impact of genetic variations on drug response, is a key area of personalized medicine. The combination of genetic data and advanced technologies will make it possible to develop more targeted drugs tailored to each individual.

- ❖ <u>Regulatory and ethical challenges</u>: The development and use of medicines require rigorous regulation to ensure their safety, efficacy and quality. However, rapid technological advances and new therapeutic models pose regulatory and ethical challenges. It is essential to put in place flexible and adapted regulatory frameworks to support innovation while protecting patient safety. In addition, protecting the confidentiality of genetic data and the responsible management of health information are becoming major issues in the field of personalized medicine.

❖ <u>Interdisciplinary collaboration</u>: In the face of these challenges and opportunities, interdisciplinary collaboration between researchers, clinicians, regulators, healthcare professionals and patients is crucial. Pooling knowledge, skills and resources will help overcome obstacles and accelerate progress in the field of pharmacology and toxicology. Communication and information exchange between the various stakeholders is essential to ensure safe and effective use of medicines and promote evidence-based practices.

Conclusion: The "Future prospects and challenges" chapter highlights promising developments in the fields of pharmacology and toxicology, as well as the challenges they face. Technological advances, personalized medicine, regulatory and ethical challenges, and interdisciplinary collaboration are all key factors that will shape the future of these disciplines. By understanding these future prospects and addressing the challenges, we can make progress towards better use of medicines and improved health for all.

16.Innovations in drug pharmacology and toxicology

Innovations in drug pharmacology and toxicology have a significant impact on drug development, efficacy and safety. These fields of research are constantly evolving, thanks to scientific and technological advances, which are improving our understanding of how drugs act on the human body and optimizing their use.

In pharmacology, many innovations have been made in the discovery and development of new drugs. Researchers have access to high-throughput screening techniques, enabling them to rapidly test thousands of chemical compounds to identify those with the potential to become new drugs. In addition, approaches such as pharmacogenomics and pharmacogenetics have emerged, enabling drug treatments to be tailored to individual genetic variations. This helps optimize efficacy and reduce adverse effects in certain patients.

Drug toxicology has also benefited from numerous innovations. Researchers use advanced techniques to assess the safety of drugs and predict their potential toxic effects. For example, in vitro methods, such as assays on human cells in culture, make it possible to assess the effects of drugs on specific cellular models. In addition, computer modeling and simulation can be used to predict drug interactions and potential toxic effects at the molecular level. These approaches reduce the need for animal experiments and speed up the process of developing new drugs.

Another major innovation concerns targeted therapies, which specifically target the molecules or biological pathways involved in disease. Thanks to a better understanding of the underlying mechanisms of disease, researchers are able to develop drugs that act more precisely and selectively. This increases the efficacy of treatments while reducing side effects. For example, targeted therapies are successfully used in the treatment of cancer, where drugs are designed to specifically inhibit the growth of cancer cells.

In addition, technological advances have enabled the development of new modes of drug delivery. For example, targeted drug delivery systems use nanotechnology to transport drugs directly to specific cells or tissues, improving efficacy and reducing adverse effects. In addition, research into drug formulations has led to developments such as sustained-release drugs, which enable less frequent administration and better therapeutic compliance.

In short, innovations in drug pharmacology and toxicology are constantly evolving, enabling the development of medicines that are more effective, safer and better adapted to individual patient needs. Thanks to the use of advanced screening techniques, computational modeling and targeted therapies, drug discovery, development and use are undergoing a significant transformation, paving the way for new possibilities in health and medicine.

17.Ethics and responsibility in drug use

Ethics and responsibility play an essential role in the use of medicines, from the point of view of healthcare professionals, patients and the pharmaceutical industry. Here are some important aspects of ethics and responsibility related to the use of medicines:

- **Equitable access**: Ethics demand that all individuals have equitable access to the medicines they need for their health. This means that medicines should not be unnecessarily restricted due to financial, geographical or socio-economic considerations. Governments, international organizations and the pharmaceutical industry have a responsibility to ensure that essential medicines are accessible to all, particularly in developing countries.

- **Accurate and transparent information**: Healthcare professionals have an ethical obligation to provide patients with accurate, comprehensive and comprehensible information on medicines, including their indications, potential side effects and available alternatives. Similarly, the pharmaceutical industry must transparently disclose the results of clinical trials and information on the safety and efficacy of medicines.

- **Informed consent**: Patients have the right to be fully informed of the potential risks and benefits of proposed medicines before giving consent for treatment. Healthcare professionals must ensure that patients understand the information provided and are able to make informed decisions about their use of medicines.

- ❖ Appropriate use : Ethics and responsibility demand that drugs be used appropriately and in line with best clinical practice. Healthcare professionals must follow established guidelines and protocols to ensure proper use of medications, avoid abuse and minimize risk to patients. Similarly, patients are responsible for following their healthcare professional's instructions and taking their medication as recommended.

- ❖ Ethical research: Drug research must meet high ethical standards, ensuring that the rights and welfare of research participants are protected. This includes obtaining informed consent, disclosing potential conflicts of interest and closely monitoring the impact of medicines on participants. Research results must be communicated transparently for the benefit of the scientific community and the public.

- ❖ Pharmaceutical industry responsibility: Pharmaceutical companies have an ethical responsibility to conduct their business in a way that respects ethical standards, the quality of medicines and patient safety. This includes conducting rigorous research, full disclosure of drug information, responsible product promotion and cooperation with regulatory authorities.

In short, ethics and responsibility are essential in the use of medicines. They ensure fair access, accurate information, informed consent, appropriate use, ethical research and accountability of the pharmaceutical industry. By adhering to these principles, we can promote the safe and ethical use of medicines, in the interests of both patients and public health.

Conclusion: Towards a better understanding of drugs and their risks

The book "Pharmacology and Toxicology of Medicines: Deciphering the Secrets of Their Effects and Risks" offers an in-depth exploration of drugs and their risks, with the ultimate aim of improving our understanding of these substances essential to human health.

Through its pages, the book plunges us into the complex world of pharmacology, revealing the mechanisms of drug action and the interactions they have with our bodies. It highlights the progress made in the discovery and development of new drugs, thanks to cutting-edge techniques such as high-throughput screening and pharmacogenomics. These advances enable us to optimize drug treatments by taking into account individual genetic variations, paving the way for more personalized and effective medicine.

The book also looks at the toxicology of drugs, highlighting the crucial importance of assessing their safety and predicting their potential adverse effects. Thanks to modern methods of toxicological evaluation, such as in vitro testing and computer modeling, we are able to identify the risks associated with drug use more quickly, and take preventive measures to minimize these risks.

Ethics and responsibility take center stage in this book, highlighting the importance of fair access to medicines, transparent and accurate information for patients, and appropriate use of treatments. Researchers, healthcare professionals and the pharmaceutical industry have a responsibility to ensure that medicines are used ethically, to the highest standards of research, clinical practice and disclosure.

In the end, "Pharmacology and Toxicology of Drugs: Deciphering the Secrets of Their Effects and Risks" reminds us that our understanding of drugs is a constantly evolving field. Thanks to scientific and technological advances, we are making progress towards a better understanding of drugs and their risks. This enables us to optimize their use, reduce adverse effects and ensure better health for all.

This book is an invaluable resource for researchers, healthcare professionals, students and anyone interested in the study of drugs and their impact on human health. It invites us to continue exploring, questioning and deepening our knowledge, with the ultimate aim of promoting the safe and informed use of medicines, for the well-being of all.

Appendix 1: Glossary

1. Pharmacology: The science of drugs, their action on the human body and their interactions with cells, tissues and organs.

2. Toxicology: The branch of pharmacology that studies the harmful effects of chemical substances on living organisms.

3. Drug: A substance used to prevent, treat or alleviate a disease or medical condition.

4. Pharmacogenomics: The study of individual genetic variations that influence an individual's response to drugs.

5. Targeted therapy: A treatment approach that specifically targets the molecules or biological pathways involved in the disease.

6. Targeted drug delivery system: A technology that transports drugs directly to specific cells or tissues, improving efficacy and reducing side effects.

7. Informed consent: The process by which a patient is fully informed of the potential risks and benefits of a treatment and gives informed consent.

Appendix 2: Index

References

1. "Goodman and Gilman's The Pharmacological Basis of Therapeutics" by Laurence L. Brunton, Bjorn C. Knollmann, Randa Hilal-Dandan.
2. "Basic & Clinical Pharmacology" by Bertram G. Katzung, Anthony J. Trevor.
3. "Principles of Pharmacology: The Pathophysiologic Basis of Drug Therapy" by David E. Golan, Armen H. Tashjian, Ehrin J. Armstrong.
4. "Rang & Dale's Pharmacology" by James M. Ritter, Rod J. Flower, Graeme Henderson.
5. "Lippincott Illustrated Reviews: Pharmacology" by Karen Whalen.
6. "Handbook of Experimental Pharmacology" by T. Kenakin, A. Christopoulos.
7. "Pharmacology: A Patient-Centered Nursing Process Approach" by Linda E. McCuistion, Kathleen Vuljoin DiMaggio, Mary Beth Winton.
8. "Lehne's Pharmacology for Nursing Care" by Jacqueline Burchum, Laura Rosenthal.
9. "Textbook of Drug Design and Discovery" by Peter M. Selzer, Yvonne Perrie, Donald P. Vis.
10. "Molecular Pharmacology: From DNA to Drug Discovery" by John Dickenson.
11. "Pharmacogenomics: Challenges and Opportunities in Therapeutic Implementation" by Sandosh Padmanabhan.
12. "Medical Pharmacology at a Glance" by Michael J. Neal.
13. "Pharmacology and Physiology for Anesthesia: Foundations and Clinical Application" by Hugh C. Hemmings, Talmage D. Egan.
14. "Pharmacology: Examination & Board Review" by Anthony J. Trevor, Bertram G. Katzung.
15. "Toxicology: Principles and Applications" by A. Wallace Hayes.
16. "Casarett & Doull's Toxicology: The Basic Science of Poisons" by Curtis D. Klaassen.
17. "Introduction to Toxicology" by John A. Timbrell.
18. "Textbook of Clinical Toxicology" by J. J. Buckley, P. D. W. Kiely.
19. "Toxicology Handbook" by Lindsay Murray, Frank Daly, Lewis Nelson.
20. "Toxicology and Clinical Pharmacology of Herbal Products" by Melanie Johns Cupp.
21. "Toxicology: A Case-Oriented Approach" by John B. Sullivan, Gary R. Krieger.
22. "Toxicology in Antiquity" by Philip Wexler.
23. "Toxicology of Organophosphate & Carbamate Compounds" by Ramesh C. Gupta.
24. "A Textbook of Modern Toxicology" by Ernest Hodgson.
25. "Handbook of Systems Pharmacology" by Uri Alon.

26. "Toxicology and Risk Assessment: Principles, Methods, and Applications" by Helmut Greim, Robert Snyder.
27. "Toxicology of the Kidney" by John H. Dirks, Sudhir V. Shah.
28. "Antibiotics: Challenges, Mechanisms, Opportunities" by Christopher Walsh.
29. "Environmental Toxicology: Biological and Health Effects of Pollutants" by Ming-Ho Yu, Emily Monosson.
30. "Toxicology: A Primer on Toxicology Principles and Applications" by Randy W. Jirtle, Frederick J. de Serres.
31. "Toxicology and Clinical Pharmacology of Herbal Products" by Melanie Johns Cupp.
32. "Anticancer Drugs: Design, Delivery, and Pharmacology" by Raphael M. Ottenbrite, Michelle A. Rudek.
33. "Handbook of Experimental Pharmacology: Antidepressants" by J. M. Monti.
34. "Introduction to Pharmacology for Nursing Students" by Dr. Venugopal K. Reddy.
35. "Pharmacology and Therapeutics for Dentistry" by Frank J. Dowd, Bart Johnson, Angelo Mariotti.
36. "Goldfrank's Toxicologic Emergencies" by Lewis R. Goldfrank, Neal E. Flomenbaum, Mary Ann Howland.
37. "Introduction to Toxicology and Food" by Tomris Altug.
38. "Pharmacology: PreTest Self-Assessment and Review" by Marshal Shlafer.
39. "Levin and O'Neal's The Diabetic Foot" by John H. Bowker, Michael A. Pfeifer.
40. "Toxicology of the Immune System: A Human Approach" by Michael I. Luster, Robert M. S. Greger.
41. "Antiviral Drugs: From Basic Discovery Through Clinical Trials" by William J. Facey, Richard L. Heel.
42. "Toxicology and Clinical Pharmacology of Herbal Products" by Melanie Johns Cupp.
43. "Handbook of Systems Pharmacology" by Uri Alon.
44. "Principles of Clinical Pharmacology" by Arthur J. Atkinson Jr, Darrell R. Abernethy, Charles E. Daniels.
45. "Toxicology: A Comprehensive Introduction" by Mark E. Stelljes.
46. "Pharmacology and Physiology for Anesthesia: Foundations and Clinical Application" by Hugh C. Hemmings, Talmage D. Egan.
47. "Toxicology of Organophosphate & Carbamate Compounds" by Ramesh C. Gupta.
48. "A Textbook of Modern Toxicology" by Ernest Hodgson.
49. "Clinical Pharmacology and Therapeutics for Veterinary Technicians" by Robert L. Bill.
50. "Environmental Toxicology: Biological and Health Effects of Pollutants" by Ming-Ho Yu, Emily Monosson.
51. "Pharmacology: Examination & Board Review" by Anthony J. Trevor, Bertram G. Katzung.

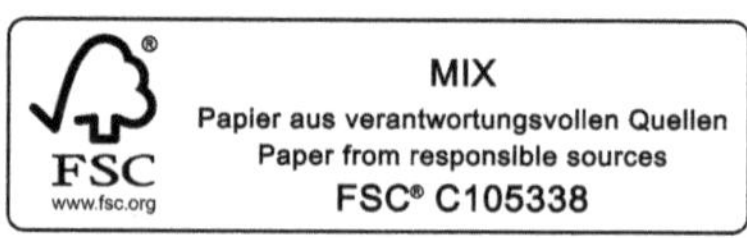

Printed by Books on Demand GmbH, Norderstedt / Germany